You can do what I did:

lose weight,

improve your health,

stay fit!

Author Manfred Popp

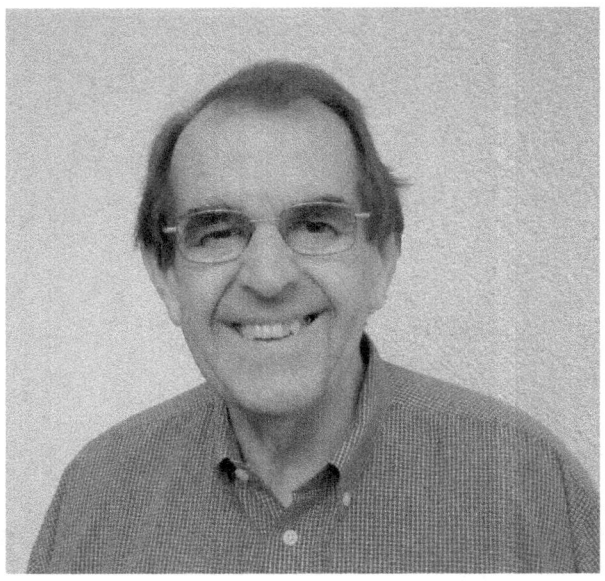

In his book the author explains, how to lose weight,
stay fit and healthy.

You can do what I did:

Lose weight,

improve your health,

stay fit!

Manfred Popp

IMPRINT

© 2014 Author Manfred Popp

Edition 1

ISBN: 978-1500580094

Printed by CreateSpace, Charleston SC, USA

Font: New Times Roman

Self-publisher: Manfred Popp, Gaimersheim 85080, Germany, Mane.Popp@t-online.de

This book is listed in the German National Bibliography, see http:/dnb.d-nb.de.

Note:

FOREWORD

This book is written for a very specific target group, the age group "60 plus", to show a way to weight loss, health and fitness. Specifically for this group of readers, I wrote this guide after practicing myself the following recommendations during the last nine years. During this time I have lost around 44 pounds of weight without dieting and without fasting. The experience gained which improved my health considerably, so I want to pass on to my senior peer group.

Manfred Popp

Table Of Contents

Personal Experience Report

In the first part of this book I am presenting my personal experience, which made me write this important topic.

Everything started in May 2005, when I decided to try to lose at least 33pounds. I did not make this decision because I wanted to look a bit better or because my clothes were getting too tight. No, it was my doctor, who made me decide, to try to improve my desolate state of health. I'll tell you in detail, how I proceeded, and, hopefully, I will prove that I was successful and that I can motivate as many seniors who are overweight as possible to implement my recommendations both with energy and motivation.

When I retired in April of 2005 from professional life, I decided to do something for my health. At that time, at the age of 64 years, although I was quite fit and had no notable health problems, my doctor was not happy with my blood pressure. As early as in 2004, he criticized my upper and lower blood pressure and said there was a borderline tendency to exceed these values. To prove his opinion he prescribed, in December 2004, an all-day blood pressure measurement, which yielded promptly as mean values of 42 measurements an upper Sys value of 160.5 and a lower slide-value of 94.0 and an average pulse of 75. Whereas, in my age group - in the words of my doctor − the normal results showed have been values from 120 to 130, slide-values between 80 and 95 and the pulse values of 60 to 90! But the averages of daily measurements were at the "top" blood pressure significantly higher and the "bottom" near the critical point, but the pulse could be considered appropriate. For me, however, it was very difficult to accept these values.

In mid 2004, I bought in a pharmacy my own blood pressure monitor for measuring at the upper arm. In the following years from mid-2004 I have made at irregular measurements intervals. The upper values were from 126 to 146, the lower ones from 79 to 92 and the pulse between 60 and 67. These lower values were not quite satisfactory, but significantly better than the upper values.

From the beginning of 2005 I began to measure my blood pressure daily, morning and evening. I stored the values in my PC, so that I got a monthly statistical survey. The monthly values, which resulted from these regular daily measurements were about "normal. These figures were self-explanatory. The "upper" level was 135 to 140, the "lower" value at around 85. Although not real substantially above the upper sys-blood pressure, the "upper" values could not satisfy me, since they were to be interpreted as average figures, and thus had a very different significance than single random measurements.

Because of this evaluation I had to recognize that my "top" blood pressure was too high on average, and also the "bottom", which is even more important than the first, in average also approached the no-go area. It was now clear to me, that I had to do something about it.

Even at the first health check as a pensioner in early May 2005 at the age of 64 years, my blood pressure was assessed as too high by the doctor. He prescribed tablets pointing out, with a slightly ironic smile, instead of the tablets I could also reduce my weight by 33 pounds, then I needed no blood pressure pills. I bought the tablets and my wife read to me at lunch with emphatic clarity the long list of side effects. It became vividly clear that I had to make a fundamental decision:

Either taking for the rest of my life pills against high blood pressure with a number of possible side effects, or reducing my weight significantly by at least 33 pounds. After an intense period of reflection I decided for losing weight.

I had to get rid of 33 pounds

I was not particularly convinced of dieting. At the age of about 30 years I had already reduced my weight by more than 40 pounds through long weeks of dieting, which was quite frustrating. This fasting was associated with a lot of loss in life quality.

And when I got back to "normal" food, the lost pounds came back and I gradually reached my former weight of around 260 pounds again. In spring 2005, my weight had stabilized between 251 pounds and 253.5 pounds, and I was trying to go down to around 218 pounds.

My goal was not only to achieve this weight loss, but the real challenge was to keep the lower weight in the long run. Therefore my action strategy did not include a crash diet. I was aware that this could mean nothing more than changing my lifestyle with the goal to maintain a lower weight in the long term.

Strategy approach to weight loss

It was therefore necessary to find promising approaches to losing weight. Generally, one assumes that a permanent weight loss is possible only after a change in eating habits and concomitant intensification of movement, which is reasonable and easy to understand. So I had to check my eating and drinking habits and to look into my sporting activities for starters. It was very evident to me that I had to change my drinking habits. For about 20 years I drank no wine, but I had got used to drink two bottles of beer every evening, or even three bottles at weekends. I saw myself thus forced to focus on the reduction of beer consumption during the evening.

Although it was not easy, I had to make, in this regard, my first major strategy decision, to drink no more beer at home, except we had guests.

As for the rest of the meal, I made a second strategic decision: to eat, in the evening, only some fruits and a low-fat portion of plain yogurt. Moreover, in future I was to have sweets only exceptionally.

Another starting point was to revise my sporting activities. In my youth I had practiced regularly, played field handball and I also did 6mile-runs. I also liked to swim, especially long distances. During my first year at Tuebingen University, I also indulged in a lot of sporting activities. But when I moved to Munich for my third semester at Munich University, my sporting enthusiasm gradually died down, partly because of the intense time-consuming study of economics, but this was surely not the only reason. Munich offered to a person from the "provinces" an incredible number of distractions. I also met my future wife, which, naturally, resulted in a shift of my interests and activities. In the following years my sportive exercises got more and more restricted, because the job took a lot of time - and in the meantime I had indeed created a family.

In 1971, I was just 30, I bought a rowing machine, with the good intention, once or twice a week, to have a fitness training. Unfortunately, however this was to remain a good intention. My professional commitments did not allow me to spare the time required for sports, so that a regular and demanding training on the rowing machine was no longer possible and I forgot about my rowing machine. My belief in doing something for my body atrophied, but not quite. I wanted, at least once a week to practice a specific endurance training, even in bad weather. That's why I bought an exercise bike and I managed, in the following years, to regularly ride it for 30 to 40 minutes once a week. After 25 years it broke down and I bought a modern machine on which I rode each weekend for 40 minutes on average.

So, at age 64, in May 2005 I could boast of some training experience on the exercise bike. therefore it was obvious to me that I should expand this endurance training selectively.

The third and perhaps most important strategy decision for the desired weight reduction, was that I decided to ride five to six times per week for about 40 to 45 minutes on my home-bike, which I had hitherto used only sporadically on weekends.

In order to achieve a "permanent weight loss of at least 33 pounds. I focused on the following goals:

- at home no more beer. Except when hosting guests
 - no more sweets
 - just yogurt and fruit for supper

- five to six times a week cycling on the exercise bike, for about 45 minutes.

It was quite clear to me that these goals represented a real challenge. To reach them I had to change my life radically, which would not be easy. However, I saw no promising alternatives.

Therefore I decided in mid-May in 2005, to adjust my future life to these aims. I was convinced that it was not enough to work along these lines only for some time until I would achieve the reduced weight, but that it would be necessary for me to orientate my future life in this sense.

LOSING WEIGHT Phase

In mid-May 2005, I began my self-chosen weight loss program.

Doing without a beer in the evening was a daily challenge, which had to be met. After the three first weeks I was able to state that serious my abstention was easier to handle very day.

Now that I drank water instead of beer in the evening, it was much easier for me to consume the daily required amount of liquid, which is particularly important. Now I was able to drink two and a half to three liters of water a day, which I could not do as a beer drinker, because beer is not one of the fluids relevant to weight loss. I had no major problems with my decision to eat only yogurt and fruit for supper. I did not renounce the rest of the food. I still had a good breakfast and adequate lunch. For lunch, my wife also laid emphasis on plenty of vegetables. Fish once a week and two to three meatless dishes alternated with various meat dishes a week. She only used vegetable oils to cook and to dress salads.

I did not feel particularly hungry, and if ever I felt life eating something, I just ate some fruit in addition. But it was particularly hard for me to do my exercise bike.

Very quickly, I realized that there was a huge difference between going by bike once a week for about 40 minutes, or making it a daily routine. It became clear to me that I simply lacked the necessary stamina. So I went over to start regular training cutting the time to 30 minutes.

The first two weeks were admittedly stressful indeed and I sweated buckets! But those two weeks went by faster than I thought and my condition had already improved.

For the next four weeks I kept on biking consistently and even increased the duration of the training units.

So the third week, I practiced up to six times per week increasing the daily cycling time from 40 to 45 minutes, while maintaining the average speed. Only on Sundays and in the holidays did I not train. By then I had progressed so far that my endurance training in the morning was really fun. At the beginning of July 2005 I felt much fitter than at the beginning of the training mid-May.

Thus it was no challenge any more for me, to do the home bike five times during the week .

Now I felt the desire in me to supplement my weekly daily training program by including an additional cardio workout. And then I remembered my old rowing machine again, that has been parked for years in a basement corner.

I decided to activate the device and to include it in my training program. I moved it to a place in the basement, where I had enough room of action. But I could only exercise on this rowing machine at the beginning in smaller time intervals, as the rowing compared to cycling was much more strenuous since it takes your whole body.

From the seventh week I did nearly 30 minutes on the bike and then I rowed for 15 minutes on the rowing machine.

Over the next four weeks, I managed to increase the rowing time continuously and by mid-August 2005, I was conditionally able to cycle regularly five to six times per week for 30 minutes and then to row another 30 minutes. And I felt very good and fit in the summer. Moreover, I could almost constantly see how my weight decreased slowly but surely!

I had made it a habit in the following years, at least five times a week in the morning to do at least for 60 minutes the endurance exercise. In the course of time, my activities focused on rowing 45 minutes on average, while I reduced cycling to about 15 to 20 minutes.

Before starting my endurance training I did a few gymnastic exercises for five to ten minutes to warm up.

To the daily endurance training including warming-up and relaxing, I added a strength training twice per week for 10 to 15 minutes with the expander and two hand weights with five kg each.

In early May 2006, about a year after my weight reducing program, I weighed an average of 233 pounds, 20 pounds less than at the beginning. That was a promising progress! This success encouraged me, to continue my program consistently.

By the end of April 2007, I weighed not more than 214 pounds, so I had lost the 37.5 pounds, I wanted to lose and even more than that! I achieved this goal without going hungry nor following any diet.

The follow-up

Now I wanted to supplement my weekly daily training program by including an additional cardio workout. I remembered my old rowing machine again that I had left standing all these years in a basement corner.

I decided to activate the device again and to include it in my training program. I put it at a place in the basement with enough operating room. But at first I could only do the rowing in smaller time intervals, as the rowing compared to cycling bike is much more strenuous.

From the seventh week on I managed to bike 30 minutes and to row for 15 minutes.

Over the next four weeks I managed to increase the rowing time continuously, and from mid-August 2005, my condition allowed me to cycle regularly five to six times per week for 30 minutes and then to row another 30 minutes. And I felt very good and fit in the summer. Moreover, I could almost constantly see how my weight decreased slowly but surely!

I had made it a habit in the following years, at least five times a week to practice in the morning for at least 60 minutes my endurance training. Gradually, my training activities shifted to rowing and the following two years I rowed 45 minutes on average, while reducing my cycling to 15 to 20 minutes.

Before starting the endurance training I had begun to do for five to ten minutes a few gymnastic exercises to warm up.

The daily endurance training with a warming-up and a relaxing phase was followed by a power training twice a week for 10 to 15 minutes with the expander and two hand weights with five kg each.

By the end of April 2007, I weighed 214 pounds, so I had reduced my excess weight by as much as 37.5 pounds! I had actually managed to surpass my original goal! And I had done it without following a diet and without going hungry.

Reducing my weight by 33 pounds

I needed about two years to achieve the desired weight loss. Now I had to try to make this weight reduction a permanent success.

This meant continuing my way consistently. I had to continue to drink no beer at home, to avoid sweets, to have only fruits for supper and go on doing my weekly endurance training.

But after practicing all that for two years, I found it, in the following years, much easier to stick to my new eating habit and to continue my physical activities. Thus in the following time, I drank no beer at home, had no sweets and ate only fruits and yogurt at supper time.

The endurance rowing and cycling on the exercise bike had become a habit. If I could not practice them a few days, I felt uncomfortable and I even felt an inner urge to use the two machines intensely. The endurance training has become normal, everyday routine and I felt deeply satisfied and it increases my physical well-being when I had completed it. I had also made it, in the two years following May 2005, a habit to swim once a week for about 30 to 45 minutes.

In the summer of 2006 I decided, to do a lot of walking, adding thus an additional component to my fitness program, regardless of the season.

In addition to walking on Sundays I had a morning walk at least three times a week of 35 to 50 minutes in the fresh air.

Since mid 2007, my movement strategy includes, on average, the following training components:

Endurance training components:

- Rowing 5 times per week for 45 minutes

- Cycling 5 times per week for 20 minutes

- Walking 3 - 4 times per week for 35 - 50 minutes

- Swimming once a week 30 - 45 minutes

Strength training:

Expander plus weights 2 times per week for 10 - 15 min

Additional gymnastic exercises to improve joint flexibility and mobility, as well as warming-up for the endurance training, 2 times per week.

To sum up, I found a perfect combination of different types of motion, which allows me not only to keep my lower weight, but which also improve my health in the long run.

I had managed to reach my aim of losing 33 pounds and to maintain this weight over a relatively long period of two years. Most of my former fat had apparently disappeared in the meantime. Moreover, my power endurance training through rowing created additional muscle mass.

Until the end of 2007 I had reduced my weight by more than 40 pounds, which clearly showed that my weight-losing strategy was not a short-time measure.

The results encouraged me to continue this strategy even further.

To obtain a comprehensive statistic of my sporting activities, I decided, in late 2007, to proceed to continuously write down records from the beginning of 2008, enabling me to evaluate the results statistically regularly.

In this way, I saw a good possibility of keeping my training under control. Each day, I was able to state how much time I invested in the various training activities.

My goal here was to practice at least 40 minutes one of the four endurance sports: walking, rowing, cycling or swimming. The only exceptions to this procedure were:

Holidays, day trips, sickness and convalescence days.

Thanks to my private statistics, I had a useful documentation at my disposal allowing me to find out the best way of achieving the desired goal.

In January 2008, I had started to write down these statistics.

Subsequent analyses showed that I had succeeded, in the first half of 2009, my daily weight loss quota, without taking into account holidays and day trips, of being physically active for 81 minutes daily. This proves that, for a senior, it is possible to be physically active throughout the week provided that he or she pass a warm-up stage in order to gain a solid physical condition. In May 2008 my weight was down to nearly 207 pounds. So I had lost about 44 pounds.

At a height of 1.83 m and an average of 94.5 kg (208.3 pounds) my body mass index (BMI) was still 28.2 ($94.5: 1,83^2$). At the beginning of May 2005 it was, however, 34, in other words, it was about 20 percent higher, which meant that it was in the area of obesity.

In May 2008, I had the opportunity to measure my weight on a body analysis scales, which indicated that the percentage of fat had gone down to 30 percent, while the muscle mass was 41.4 percent. Since muscles are heavier than fat, however, my BMI in May 2008 may not necessarily hinted to obesity.

With regard to the desired weight reduction I can boast of a weight loss of 44 pounds.

From 2009 to 2013, that is over a period of 4 years, my program consistently, both in terms of diet, as well as the exercise program.

Both, the endurance exercises in my own home, as well as the regular outdoor walking had become a normal routine for me.

In this time, I succeeded in walking 3 − 4 times a week for not less than 45 minutes throughout the year, except for days of illness or day trips. I also managed to do endurance exercises for at least 45 minutes at an average of five days a week. These exercises included home rowing, home biking on a bicycle ergometer, walking on a step machine and swimming. My goal was always, to stretch outdoor walking and cardio training over the week so, that I was active for 30 minutes on each day of the week, except for holidays, illness, convalescence days and day trips.

In 2009, I managed to practice that training program consecutively, with the exception of only three days!

Results after nine years

The results after eight years are very promising!

My weight

9 years ago

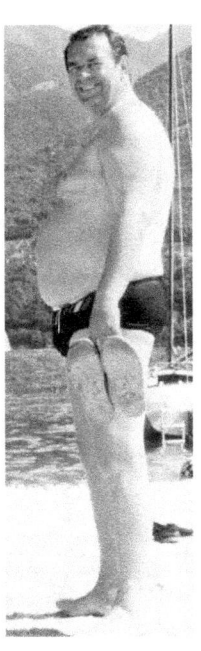
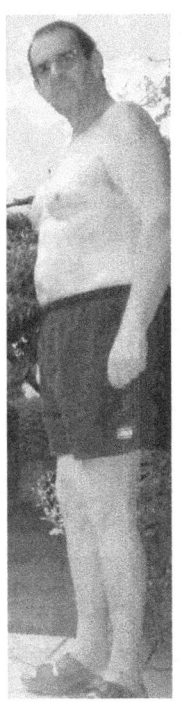

The right photo dates from the summer of 2008 after three years of carrying out my slimming program! The pictures from before starting and after finishing the program speak for themselves. In summer 2014 I was 73 years of age, so that it made sense for me at this time to draw a balance-sheet.

My weight was meanwhile at around 209.5 pounds, in other words, the scale shows nearly 44 pounds less than at the beginning of my weight efforts concept in May 2005.

Fitness report

At the age of 73 years, my fitness is much better than 10 years ago. This is certainly due to regularly performed sports activities, which I indulged in: the endurance training on the rowing machine and the bicycle ergometer. Since I practiced this training with growing intensity over the years, it had a very beneficial effect on my physical condition. It is no longer hard on me, to regularly exercise at least five days a week for about 60 minutes. It seems, on the contrary, that my body requires this training now that it is in full swing.

Effects on blood pressure and pulse

How has this weight loss affected my blood pressure?

It was precisely my physician-assessed high blood pressure that had led me to reduce my weight so that I would not have to rely on blood pressure reducing medication. Doctors generally consider weight loss to be essential for maintaining health. And in retrospect, I can only agree with this assessment after completing this eight-year action program I have been fit and healthy.

In April and May 2008, I had measured my blood pressure and pulse again pretty regularly every morning. I compared the measured values with the average values of 2004 and 2005.

The figures clearly showed that the reduction of my body weight actually led to a significant improvement of blood pressure and pulse. The average April / May 2008 value of the upper blood pressure was 123, and had decreased by almost 9 percent, while the lower value of 85 in 2004, had fallen to 77 in 2008 and therefore was by nearly 9.5 percent lower than before the start of my weight reduction program. All values were already at that time located largely within the normal range and the statement of my family doctor "33 pounds less and you do not need blood pressure pills" had been fully confirmed.

This positive development was visible in the values that I measured from January to April in 2010.

Blood pressure / pulse

Date	upper value	lower value	pulse
01/22/10	114	72	59
01/27/10	132	80	54
01/28/10	132	80	47
01/29/10	125	74	57
01/30/10	117	77	56
02/03/10	126	82	54
02/04/10	138	79	54
02/05/10	123	73	50
02/06/10	114	70	51
02/08/10	125	68	63
02/09/10	117	71	53
02/12/10	119	73	53
02/14/10	124	68	57
02/16/10	125	68	59
02/17/10	115	71	53
02/20/10	127	71	58
02/21/10	133	74	49
02/22/10	116	74	55
02/23/10	125	77	55

02/25/10	118	74	53
02/26/10	123	76	59
02/27/10	127	77	51
02/28/10	127	72	51
03/02/10	125	70	61
03/04/10	129	74	50
03/05/10	119	71	52
03/06/10	128	75	52
03/10/10	119	76	51
03/11/10	128	74	53
03/12/10	123	72	52
03/13/10	115	72	55
03/14/10	128	72	52
03/16/10	114	69	52
03/18/10	126	73	55
03/22/10	117	62	49
03/23/10	111	71	57
03/24/10	119	82	50
03/30/10	126	73	54
03/31/10	122	81	51
04/01/10	117	72	53
04/03/10	124	76	53
04/06/10	122	80	54
04/08/10	122	70	54
04/10/10	117	75	52
04/11/10	123	72	57
04/12/10	128	76	57
12/30/99	128	80	52
04/15/10	124	73	54
04/17/10	118	73	53

Average 2010 123	**74**	**54**
Average 2004 135 **Second half-year**	85	63

The positive effect of regular endurance exercise is most clearly shown by reduction of the pulse: The original value of 63 beats per minute in 2004 declined to 54 beats in 2010.

Effect on blood sugar

It is often said that endurance training has a positive effect on blood sugar levels. The corresponding "glucose" parameter was expected to be lower than 100 in the blood analysis.

In the springs of 2006, 2007, 2008 and 2010, I measured the corresponding values and found the following results: 80 mg / dl in 2006, 85 in 2007, 78 in May 2008 and 89 in May 2010.

Effect on blood values

As part of the health check my blood values have shown a generally positive trend, which were also due to the beneficial efforts of my program.

Cholesterol values have a special significance for human health. The corresponding value CHOL in the laboratory evaluation at 140 - 220 md / dl is viewed by doctors as normal. In the years 2007, 2008 and 2010, my cholesterol level was regularly at 195, which is within in the normal range.

According to the physicians' assessment cholesterol may cause deposits on the vessel walls and therefore cause arterial obstruction. It is considered a risk factor for cardiovascular diseases such as heart attack and stroke. We distinguish between HDL and LDL cholesterol. Especially an elevated LDL level is dangerous, according to medical research results. It can occur due to constant fatty food. A healthy diet rich in fruits, vegetables and fish, which contains many unsaturated fatty acids, should, on the other hand, increase the positive HDL. Particular importance is attached to the ratio between HDL and LDL. A ratio of 2.9 is considered to be the desired value.

Health effects

Regarding my overall health situation I can confirm, after eight years of trying, that my condition has shown a very positive development. In the period before 2005, I always had bronchial problems and from time to time I suffered from bronchial catarrhs. From spring to late summer, I was pretty regularly hit by severe allergy attacks, so that I often could not go outside for a long time despite allergy tablets.

Three to four times a year, I had severe pain in the right ankle, which incapacitated me two to three days and kept me from moving. Several times a year I suffered from colds and recurring bladder infections.

Now at age 73 I can say, in retrospect, that my general well-being has improved fundamentally.

- I have no more bronchial problems.

- In the last four years I've had no more allergic attacks.

- The pain in my ankle has disappeared.

This positive development is clearly a result of the health program I practiced all these years! The consistent implementation of this program is thus not only associated with a permanent weight loss in old age, but also has a very obvious positive impact on my overall well-being! Besides, on top of an improved well-being through targeted endurance training and walking in the fresh air the immune system is generally strengthened.

Conclusion

In summer 2014, after the completion of my 73nd year of life, I can state, after eight years of fitness training, the following results:

- I have lost approximately 44 pounds.
- My blood pressure readings are stable in the "healthy" range: in June 2013 my upper blood pressure is 120 - 130 and my lower blood pressure is 70 - 75.
- My pulse is at 53-60 per minute. My blood sugar level is also positive nearly 90.
- My general health condition has improved considerably.
- My physical condition is much better than before. All in all, the program I realized during the last eight years has been very successful! I have achieved not only an important loss of weight, but also a desired reduction of my blood pressure.

It is in my view a procedural concept that is perfectly suited to bring about an effective long-term reduction in body weight and a targeted improvement of blood pressure levels and obviously of blood sugar levels. I am convinced that this is, particularly for older people, of vital importance. Just for seniors there is a risk of accumulating weight and, therefore, of being confronted with increased blood pressure and blood sugar values. Moreover, it is a fact, that increasing age due to diminishing physical fitness and strength, the risk of injuries and other disabilities become more likely. This can only be softened by appropriate training measures.

After eight years of training I can tell with conviction that this training concept has a consistently positive impact, especially for seniors "60 plus", that is for seniors to my own age group.

Another important side effect reacting from a lower body weight is that both blood pressure and blood sugar can also be improved. My own values in this respect prove that this is possible.

Thus the implementation of the recommended program can significantly improve the overall general physical well-being.

My personal experience encouraged me to formulate these recommendations, which, I am convinced, will lay the foundations for a healthy life in old age.

"How to stay fit and healthy"

A GUIDE FOR SENIORS

Of course, the following suggestions cannot guarantee you'll stay in good health when you are old! And in the case of a specific disease, elderly people must consult a doctor. But our well-being is to a large extent in our own hands if we behave responsibly.

What is most important for the success of our program is that you are really willing to implement it consistently and regularly for the rest of your life! And now, have a good go at it. Go ahead without delay in accordance with our recommendations concerning the improvement of your lifestyle.

It is up to you to assess the time you may require to carry out your exercise program. Unlike professional people, senior citizens will find it particularly suitable because they will find plenty of time to follow our proposals.

All the following recommendations are based on the experience I made over the last nine years. I am writing this at the age of 73. So you see I am a senior myself!

Before starting the exercise program you should consult your doctor to confirm that nothing stands in the way. This is particularly important for your endurance training.

The guide includes several stages, and good overall results are conceivable only through the interaction of the various parts of the program.

I attach special importance, however, to the dietary hints, ensuring the enhancement of your immune system and to the details concerning the endurance training!

Recommendation Number ONE - quit smoking

If you are 60 years old and you are still smoking you must stop smoking as soon as possible. Of course it is not easy to stop smoking, but there are many seniors who are no longer addicted to tobacco!

As far as I am concerned I decided to stop smoking at age 40, although I was a heavy smoker, who smoked up to 20 cigarettes a day.

It took me four attempts at giving up smoking before I managed to get away from nicotine at age 42! Now, in 2014, that I am 73, I am very glad that I managed to stop smoking for good.

I am absolutely convinced that an elderly smoker's health is continuously at risk. Any doctor can underline this fact on the base of an instant diagnosis! Therefore giving up smoking for good is an absolute must.

By the way this recommendation is, of course, also relevant for younger people, since use of nicotine is harmful for everybody.

To cut a long story short: Forget about any attempt at improving your well-being if you can't refrain from smoking!

Recommendation Number TWO - reduce your weight

If you are overweight read the following:

Statistically, there is a great number of elderly people, who are overweight.

Obesity is certainly one of the negative side effects of today's affluent society. Obesity causes a number of health risks.

I can state that my blood pressure achieved good results when I started losing weight. We all know that high blood pressure is a big health threat for the elderly.

Many doctors believe Type II diabetes is mainly caused by obesity. So, don't hesitate and declare war on overweight!

In addition to high blood pressure and diabetes, and apart from the medical perspective there are a number of arguments speaking in favor of doing away with obesity.

In addition to the overweight factor, in recent years, the body fat factor, has become an important indicator. Nutrition experts agree that the percentage of body fat of the overall weight should not exceed 23% for men and 27% for women. They point out that the proportion of body fat increases while the muscle mass decreases at the same time, and this applies for both sexes.

An excessive percentage of body fat is, according to the current medical expertise, associated with high blood pressure, high cholesterol values and promotes heart disease, diabetes mellitus, gastrointestinal disorders and even some cancers.

Men, as statistics show are more often confronted with overweight problems than women: their body fat causes very often a large abdominal volume. And it is this belly fat that medical experts consider particularly dangerous, because abdominal cells permanently hand over this fat to the bloodstream. According to the experts, the human body has to produce cholesterol to facilitate the circulation of this fat, which leads to an excessive cholesterol level and therefore increases the risk of cardiovascular troubles.

Many seniors have to deal with problems resulting from overweight-, because they are far from what is considered to be their normal weight.

To determine the degree of obesity as compared to what should be one's normal weight, we must refer to the Body Mass Index (BMI) The BMI of a person follows the formula = weight (kg): height (m) ^{2} in the metric system. In the internet you 'll find formulas that allow in feet, inches and pounds. This method is not agreed upon by of all the experts, because it does not distinguish between fat and muscle mass, muscle mass is heavier than fat, however. An athletic type can therefore have a relatively high BMI without being overweight. But for your health needs, the BMI suffices as a guide line for assessing the degree of your obesity.

We distinguish the following main weight categories:

Category	BMI (kg/m^2)
underweight	under 18.5
normal weight	18,5 - 24,9
overweight	25 - 29,9
obesity (adiposity)	over 30

In addition, it is recommended to measure your waist line, as this reflects the degree to which the body fat must be considered to be a health risk. A waistline of 34.7 inches for women and 40.2 inches for men should not be exceeded.

But even without any measuring and BMI calculations most seniors will know whether they bring too much weight on the scale.

When you are getting older the probability of putting on weight increases. A quiet life, the lack of professional or educational stress, a rather comfortable way of living, all these factors are connected with the risk of putting on weight.

I am convinced that an effective long-term weight loss is feasible only by changing one's eating and drinking habits, along with simultaneous efficient training activities.

In this context I would like to point out that adjusting nutritional habits should not be conceived only in terms of dieting. Empirical studies show that going on a diet is, more often than not, counterproductive.

Dieting does not foster a marked reduction in body fat, for the body loses water first and muscle mass thereafter. That means that the percentage of body fat increases as a result of going on a diet. However, the higher the fat content, the lower is, after a diet, the loss in energy consumption, because fat tissue requires significantly less energy than muscle tissue. As a result, you are, after a diet, worse off than before, since the loss of muscle tissue deteriorates the fat burning and thus the consumption of calories is permanently lower than before the diet.

In the following let us talk about what can be done about slimming down a bit. The corresponding headings are "nutritional adjustment" and "physical endurance training".

Recommendation Number THREE – changing your eating habits

Nutrition wise your general goal must be to reduce your daily amount of calories per day. But let's achieve this goal without you having to go hungry all the time while you definitely reduce your need in calories, which at the same time results in a definite loss of body weight.

On the other hand, of course, you must keep a reasonable balance as far as blood sugar and cholesterol levels and other blood parameters are concerned. Especially elderly people run a health risk if their diet is too fat.

My good blood test results are due to the fact that, in the last nine years, I consistently changed my eating and drinking habits. The following advice presupposes a long-term program.

REDUCE your ALCOHOL consumption

Cut down your beer and wine consumption.

This does not mean that you have to dispense with it totally! But, according to my doctor beer or wine are ultimately converted into fat by the body, which should be avoided if you want to stick to your health concept. In addition, your liver and kidneys will appreciate your decision to drink less alcohol! A glass of red wine or one bottle of beer a day, however, are acceptable in my doctor's opinion.

Instead, drink plenty of water from the tap or mineral water; for it is of absolute importance for us seniors to drink plenty of water. You should drink at least two liters a day, in addition to coffee or tea.

REDUCE your MEAT consumption

Don't eat meat more than three times a week, poultry excepted. Make once a week your main dish a mixed tomato-cucumber-paprika-onion salad, if need be supplemented by some feta cheese.

Red vegetables such as tomatoes, peppers, and others are particularly healthy. Once or twice per week, you should eat fish. Fish contains important health omega-3 fatty acids. Such diet will also keep you mentally fit. You may eat lots of vegetables and salads. Use vegetable oils only and just a tad of salt. If you focus on eating "red" meat, you reduce your cholesterol levels, and moreover, this diet has a favorable effect on your body weight.

Further recommendations

Have fruit for supper

In the evening; you should eat only fruit, accompanied by low-fat yogurt, possibly mixed with oatmeal or cereal. It makes sense to stick to a kind of fruit, for example, an apple and a pear, that is available more or less throughout the year. If you add to these fruits a seasonal type of fruit, you will always have a varied evening meal.

Improve your breakfast habits

Banish sausage, meat and cheese from the breakfast table and rather use curds instead of butter or margarine half the time.

Avoid sweets

In other words, reduce sugar consumption. Avoid sweets like chocolate, chocolates, cream cakes, pastries and whipped cream.

The above recommendations are meant to reduce the consumption of fats, thus curbing obesity and blood values At the same time, however, a one-sided diet must be avoided. In any case, the human body must be adequately supplied with all the necessary nutrients, minerals and vitamins. Precisely for this reason vegetables and fruit take an important place in my daily diet. Meat consumption must be restricted. As for sausages, my wife and I excluded them entirely from our shopping list, as well as fat cheese, which comes only on certain holidays on the table. In my opinion, the food I recommend includes an all-round supply of all essential nutritional components.

Recommendation Number FOUR – strengthening the immune system

Our immune system protects our body from foreign, harmful pathogens such as viruses and bacteria, and also recognizes and fights the body's own degenerated cells.

Developing a robust immune system is, especially for us seniors, very significant. It largely determines whether we can mobilize enough defense power against diseases. The better this immune system works, the more independent we seniors are of tablets and medicine.

We seniors have - in contrast to most working people - the advantage of being no longer constrained to work long hours professionally.

Thus, we can sleep long enough, even if we went to bed late in the night. Thanks to longer sleep cycles - sleep experts recommend seven hours - our body can recover sufficiently and therefore regenerate. Thus our immune system can recover particularly well, because many immune-active substances are released, which increase the protective powers of the immune system. In this regard we seniors are at an obvious advantage.

It is known that vitamins, trace elements and minerals strengthen the human immune system. Certain vitamins can fight off aggressive free radicals, which damage cells and weaken the immune system.

Therefore, a balanced diet providing for sufficient vitamins, minerals and trace elements, corresponding to the structure described in the above "diet" recommendation, is particularly important for the stabilization of the immune system.

In this context, arises the issue of so called "food supplements" an issue, which is being repeatedly discussed. Here, I can often hear the argument that a balanced diet with lots of vegetables, salads and fruit can be viewed as an adequate supply of vitamins. But nevertheless, there is, in my opinion, no absolute impediment to consuming certain additional diet supplements. Especially for us seniors, I personally believe it can be useful to take to specific vitamins and trace elements in the form of tablets or capsules. During the "cold" months my wife and I, for example, take one capsule daily with vitamin C and the trace element zinc. We also take, throughout the year, tablets or pills containing mineral calcium and vitamin E. In recent years, we have also ingested for four to six weeks a daily quantum of the trace element selenium tablets in relatively small doses. Adequate selenium supply is reputed among experts as being particularly important for a properly functioning immune system.

In my opinion, as a general rule, for older people, it is preferable to take rather more than not enough food supplements.

On the base of my own experiences, there are two further ways to positively influence the immune system of elderly people.

Walking

I recommend walking for seniors in particular. Walking in the fresh air is particularly important because it provides the whole body with oxygen, which is of real importance for senior citizens. Fresh air also promotes the blood flow to the mucous membranes of the respiratory tract, repelling thus cold viruses more easily. Moreover, health experts assert that moving in fresh air also strengthens the immune system directly: It makes for more immune cells.

In addition, joints, tendons and muscles are not particularly stressed and there is no significant risk of falling. The sense of balance and coordination skills are also promoted. Since women and men have only two legs for walking, their regular workout is for seniors particularly important ensuring thus the ability to walk well as long as possible.

Under the influence of the sunlight UV-B radiation the body creates in the skin itself vitamin D, which is considered by physicians as particularly beneficent for human health.

Therefore, I recommend, as a first measure to strengthen the immune system, an average of four weekly outdoor walks of 40 to 60 minutes. This should be done throughout the year, whatever the weather is like. When it rains or snows, breathable, wind-and rain-repellent clothing is imperious. Cotton underwear is not suitable, because it increases transpiration and thus runs the risk of hypothermia.

When the sun shines, on the other hand it is recommendable to wear appropriately woven garments and sunglasses to block UV radiation, and to apply a sun cream or sunblock

Sauna

Taking a sauna not only peps up the human vascular system, but also invigorates the body and probably also strengthens the immune system. A sauna session with at least three sauna-visits, each followed by intensive cooling under the cold shower or in the plunge pool with a corresponding period of rest and relaxation is good for our health and contributes to our mental well-being.

Since my thirtieth year I have been taking saunas regularly, and I wouldn't like to stop doing that. I am convinced that going for a sauna once a week is very beneficial to the immune system.

Recommendation Number FIVE – strengthening the physical condition

We seniors will only be in good physical shape if we begin to care deliberately and continuously for our health.

In addition to doing gymnastic exercises for the elderly we should focus on a largely stress-free strength training.

Before, however, talking about gymnastics and strength training in more detail, I should like to point out how our general day routine can be structured to improve our physical condition.

It is generally recommended to walk up the stairs instead of taking the elevator and to do errands on foot instead of driving the car. But even when you watch television you can do something for your body: Sit down for a short time, not in an armchair, but on a stool. Now stand up, 10 to 20 times slowly. If you do this exercise regularly, you strengthen the entire leg muscles.

Take, while television watching, a water bottle, filled with at least 0.5 liter of water and hold this bottle in your right hand with your arm outstretched, and then switch over to your left arm, and that as long as you can in each case.

Take two hand clamps and keep them compressed for few minutes while you are watching evening news on TV. This will positively invigorate your hand and forearm muscles in the long run.

At the beginning of 2010, my wife purchased a Pilates ball with a small diameter, on which she regularly bobs up and down to strengthen her pelvis. Such an exercise, which takes about 5 – 10 minutes, is an excellent way of strengthening not only leg and thigh muscles, but also the internal abdominal muscles. In addition to this, in the long run, it also prevents hemorrhoids! Such daily exercises have a beneficial effect not only on seniors, but also on juniors.

Gymnastics

The following recommendations are important for several reasons.

They invigorate the entire body and stabilize your fitness.

Secondly, such exercises promote your physical flexibility, which for seniors, is of particular importance.

They also enhance your sense of balance.

To achieve these goals, I suggest exercises for which you will need about 15 to 20 minutes two to three times per week.

The more often you do these gymnastic exercises, the more advantageous will your physical overall condition be affected, and the fitter you get, the easier it will be for you, to maintain your sense of balance in your everyday life.

Power Training

The recommendations for strength training are intended to mainly pursue the following purposes:

Preventing a possible muscle failure. Time and again, you can learn in the media that from age 30 you start losing muscle power, and when you are 80, you will have lost up to 25 percent of your former muscular strength. This should be a warning to the 60 plus generation!

The following training equipment is to be recommended:

An expander and two 11 pound hand weights.

Both types of devices are easily obtainable at reasonable prices in specific shops or via the internet.

I recommend strength training for 10 to 15 minutes at least twice, better three times per week. The goal is to achieve a significant strengthening of arm, chest and back muscles, which will have a positive effect on your general physical condition. In addition, joints, tendons and bones in the area of the upper body will also benefit from this muscle training. This kind of power training will specifically work against the dangerous loss of muscular strength, which, in my eyes, is especially important! It is certainly not possible to prevent this loss of strength entirely when you get older, but it is up to us seniors to slow down this process.

Recommendation number SIX - endurance training as basis for fitness and health

I personally give a very high priority to endurance training, because it certainly is not only profitable to your physical fitness and stamina. It has a positive influence on the overall physical well-being, as it effectively improves blood pressure levels and also appears to have favorable effect on blood sugar.

It also obviously keeps young! In the PHARMACY Newspaper of 15 November 2009 the following statement can be read: "The fact that sport has a positive effect on health, show many studies. Now a study from the Universities of Saarbruecken and Homburg in Germany says, that intense endurance training delays the aging process of certain cells. Among other things, it has an effect on the so-called telomeres in white blood cells. Telomeres are the ends of the chromosomes. They become shorter with each cell division until they eventually no longer function and the cell perishes. Endurance training seems to help ensure that the telomeres are better protected from degradation and aging of the cells is more slowly." This promising fact alone should make us seniors concentrate on a specific endurance training!

Before starting to give some important training recommendations, let me give you a piece of advice: before starting endurance training over a period of at least three to four weeks you should daily check your blood pressure and pulse, preferably at the same time of day and thus establish a record of your values. If you do not have a blood pressure monitor, yet you should buy one. You should choose a blood pressure gage, which can be applied to your upper arm.

If you have written down your daily values to determine appropriate averages for a sufficiently long period of time, you can later, after having carried out the recommended program, correspondingly compare these important health data with the original values. And you will see, that these values will have a positive downward trend. This will encourage you to continue the program!

These initial values of blood pressure and pulse, possibly supplemented by the blood glucose level, are the basic data that will allow you later to control your success progress.

Suitable endurance sports for elderly persons

There are several sports, which can be practiced by everybody, such as jogging, cycling, swimming.

These endurance sports can be carried out without overburdening the heart rate, but allowing fat burning optimally.

Elderly people must make sure that they do not overstrain joints, tendons and muscles, and keep their balance. They should consult their doctor accordingly.

Jogging

By jogging the joints are particularly affected (3 - to 7-times the corresponding body weight according to experts) and also the latent danger of falling – especially for seniors – cannot be excluded, I can recommend this particular endurance sport only conditionally for older people.

Personally, I have begun mid-2009, four years after starting my program, to jog the last 15 to 20 minutes of regular walking. I noted with pleasure that I had no problems with the joints and my condition was all right.

However, from late spring to fall, I limited the jogging, so that I only walked in the cold season. In the winter, the risk of falling while jogging is, for the elderly, relatively large, so in my eyes, this endurance sport is not particularly suited as a year-long-endurance sport for seniors, although jogging is certainly very beneficial to health.

In addition, seniors should, as long as they have excess weight, refrain from jogging to avoid greater stress in the joints and tendons.

This group of seniors should focus on regular walking, because walking will also increase without doubt the stamina. Only when, after two or three years, the weight has been reduced accordingly, and a good general condition is given, these seniors can take up a little jogging.

Outdoor Biking

The goal of the endurance training is to move mainly regularly throughout the year, so that the resulting beneficial effects on health and fitness prevail.

This means that outdoor cycling does not apply because it cannot be practiced throughout the year due to weather conditions. However if the weather is fine occasional biking is highly recommendable to improve balance and coordination skills.

Swimming

Swimming is also one of the health promoting sports and can also be carried out as an endurance sport.

Body weight plays only a minor role and it strengthens virtually most of the muscles.

If swimming is to have a positive effect on fitness and health, it must be practiced several times a week throughout the year. I recommend to everybody who can swim, to swim as regularly as possible once a week. Try to swim if possible for 30 minutes in a row.

Appropriate sports equipment for

endurance training

Especially suitable for seniors to increase stamina is cycling on a **bicycle ergometer**. Cycling serves, mainly to strengthen the leg and buttock muscles.

In addition, to the training on the exercise bike I recommend riding on a **home rowing machine**!

Rowing activates all major muscle groups of the body and strengthens, in particular, back and shoulder muscles, arm muscles, leg muscles, stomach and buttocks.

Both endurance sports improve the oxygen absorption, which has a beneficial health effect for seniors.

Another device, a **stepper** is well suited for seniors as a training tool for endurance sports. Pedaling on such a stepper will not only train the leg and buttock muscles, but also the hip joints will be subjected to a healthy workout. In addition, this training has a very positive effect on the sense of balance of seniors!

The exercise time should be at least 15 to 20 minutes, which should not be a problem, since this unit is not very strenuous. In about 20 minutes of training, however, only about 85 calories are consumed.

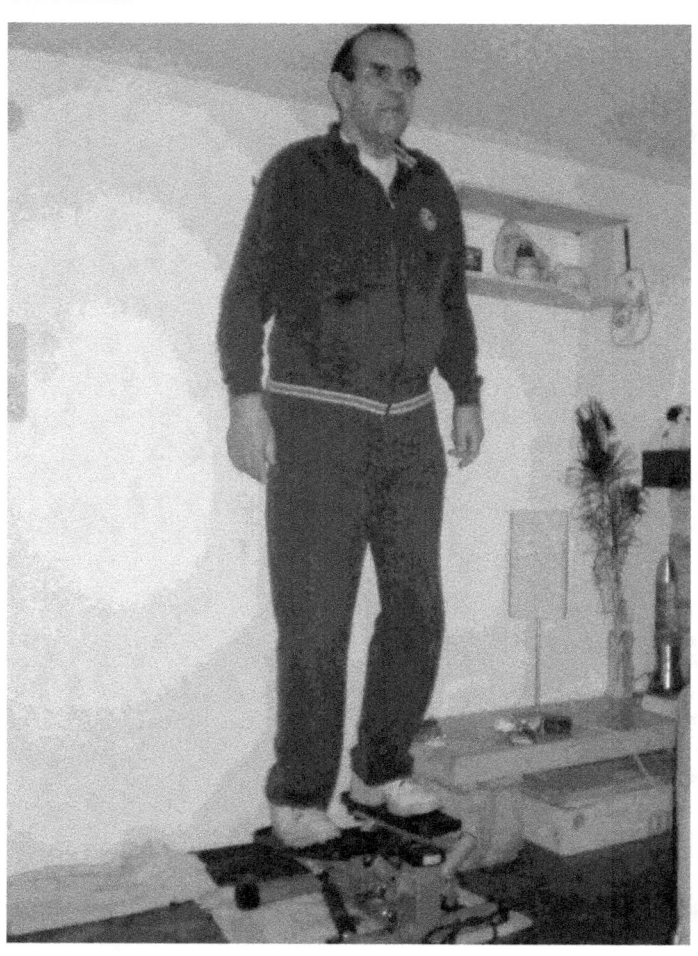

The stepper has the advantage that it requires less space and no major expense. There are no particular installation problems. Therefore I recommend a purchase!

Concerning the recommended training on exercise bike or bicycle ergometer and on a rowing machine also sets the question, whether we should do this in one of the many fitness centers.

Of course, probably all center offer to train on these two devices.

However, it is not very motivating for an older man or woman, to train on one of the cardio machines alongside mostly young, athletic types, for where everyone can see you.

In this regard, everybody has to make his own decision, whether he goes to a studio, or rather acquires the devices for home training. Not only financial aspects play a role, but it is also a question of logistics. Personally, It would take me at least 15 to 20 minutes by car to get to the next fitness center, if road conditions are normal. To gain time I have decided to carry out the training in my own home.

Accordingly, I recommend to purchase the two devices needed for the endurance training and to find a suitable space for them at home. I put the exercise bike in the bedroom and the rower in the basement, which is well ventilated.

Based on my personal experiences with both devices, I can say with conviction that the presence of both training units in one's own home is necessary if you want to do your training every day , so that you are totally independent of external weather conditions.

Additional advice

In addition to the acquisition of the two endurance sport machines, I think the purchase of a heart rate measuring tape and a matching pulse clock are particularly important, because without measuring his heart rate a senior should not practice endurance sports.

Devices with chest strap systems are preferable because they are also suitable for the rowing machine, if it is equipped with an LCD display and pulse reception, the pulse on the device display can be monitored, which is of particular importance for seniors.

Only a pulse measurement system allows the training intensity endurance sports to monitor continuously ensuring that no excessive training is practiced. Excessive training can be dangerous.

One method to determine the correct intensity of training is based on the so-called "maximum heart rate" MHR.

This is a formula, which is the result of years of sports medicine research. It reads:

Maximum heart rate = 220 - age.

Five training units can be distinguished, each playing a specific role as to the intensity of aerobic exercise.

These five areas of training divide up as follows:

Units	MHR
Health zone (fitness / health stability):	50 - 60%
Fat burning (active metabolism):	60 - 70%
Aerobic Zone (fitness improvement):	70 - 80%
Anaerobic Zone:	80 - 90%
Warning Zone (top limit):	90 - 100%

The health zone requires long, but slow, easy and low-stress intensity endurance exercises. This zone should be used by beginners or those with low fitness. It will also be used by experts for pre-exercise warming up.

The fat burning phase during an aerobic exercise will strengthen your heart, as well as optimize the burning of fat, because during this process the energy mainly comes from body fat and less from carbohydrates. An active metabolism, and thus the long term training effect in terms of weight reduction, is achieved as a result of an endurance exercise at 60 - 70% of the personal maximum heart rate. It must be mentioned here that in this phase the pounds are not faster reduced than in the other units, because only the calorie balance is responsible for weight loss.

In this context I would like to mention the following points: As far as calorie supply is concerned, many people think in terms of kilocalories (kcal). But many cardio machines with electronic scoring specify the calories in kilojoules (kJ). The following conversion formula applies in this case: 1 kilocalorie (kcal) is equivalent to 4.1868 kilojoules (kJ) or 1 kilojoule (kJ) corresponds to 0.2388 kilocalorie (kcal). When I practice on my bicycle ergometer for 45 minutes producing 100 to 110 watts, then the display shows, that I have a calorie consumption of about 1600 kilojoules, which corresponds only to roughly 380 calories. Therefore, the same unit is necessary at both sides of the caloric balance.

The following table shows examples for from 64 to 68 years of age with the corresponding heart rate values for the five units:

Training Area	Heart rate	64 years pulse	66 years pulse	68 years pulse
health area	50-60	78 - 94	77 - 92	76 - 91
fat loss area	60-70	95 - 109	93 - 107	92 - 106
aerobic area	70-80	110 - 125	108 - 123	107-122
anaerobic a.	80-90	126 - 140	124 - 138	123-137
warning area	90-100	141 - 156	139 - 154	138-152

There is of course no formula individually applicable with absolute accuracy! The above mentioned data must be regarded as average values and they have therefore to be interpreted as a well-meant piece of advice.

As endurance sports cycling and rowing are recommendable, primarily as a longer term training to lose fat.

But before discussing these two types of endurance more closely, I should like to give a number of hints.

Exercise bikes are probably found in many households. This unit does not require any additional advice. If such a bike is not available, you can easily get in any sporting goods store a good overview of the different offers.

You will have to choose between an exercise home bike and a stationary ergometer bike. While with the cheaper exercise home bikes the pedal resistance is generally controlled manually via a specific, limited number of resistance levels, an ergometer, which is connected to the mains supply, usually allows for highly variable wattages.

The most important advantages of the ergometer. are the individually adjustability of the resistance level and its support through flexible IT programs.

However, it is not absolutely necessary to decide for a technically complex system solution, which is quite costly. It is only important, that you will use the home bike regularly!

In regard of the rowing machine it is necessary to define more in detail what is desirable so that you have a clear idea of what you really need. Not all sports shops have such equipment ready to show. Moreover, the price range from cheap to very expensive is particularly large.

Let me give you a few hints to facilitate your decision: It is important that the device has a very high number of selectable resistance levels.

Besides, the LCD screen should show above all the pulse measurement with the help of a cardio belt.

It is also important that the rowing machine include a possible high weight capacity (because of your own weight).

In view of the motions there are for the rowers two different technical solutions: on the one side those with bracket arms, with correct rowing arms. These devices provide an oar handle for each hand. Here the movement corresponds to that of a "real" rowing boat. To implement this, hydraulic cylinders are placed in the rowing arms as a braking system, which produce the resistance during the backward movement. On the other hand, units are available with a cable, which is drawn with both hands with the help of a handle. Here also many other brake systems in usage, for example, the magnetic brake system or the air resistance system.

The first category represents, as a rule, the cheaper solutions than the latter group of devices. However, you can safely row on both systems and everybody must decide how much money he is willing to spend.

As for as I am concerned, I have purchased my new rowing machine from a discounter.

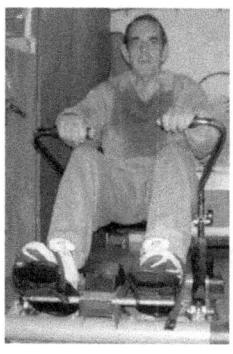

What I like about my device, is especially the almost infinite adjustability of the hydraulic control of the resistance of the rowing arms almost infinitely. So I am in a position to adjust the rowing resistance in the course of time to my training progress. Training on the rowing machine is surely an excellent endurance exercise, making at the same time for strength training.

Recommendations for working with the cycling coach and the rowing machine

Using the rowing machine is surely an excellent aerobic exercise, which at the same time, results in strength training, provided that the resistance is adjusted correspondingly. But even if the rudder resistance is operated in a low level, arm and leg muscles are pretty well strengthened. Therefore, untrained elderly persons will show signs of fatigue relatively quickly. Based on my own experience, therefore I recommend that this target group practice the endurance training on these two devices in different stages.

Start the first endurance training cycling on the bike ergometer in the first four weeks six days a week for 20 minutes, always with chest strap and heart rate monitor.

Initially set the pedaling resistance or the wattage at a level so that the 20 minutes in the first two weeks don't affect the health zone in accordance with the pulse measurement. This means that, for example, your pulse should move between about 76 and 94 beats per minute, if you are 64 to 68 years old.

From the third week you increase your pedaling speed adding a bit more resistance so that your pulse gradually reaches the area of fat loss. You should then have arrived at an average speed of about 15.5 miles / hour. This will, very likely, result in a fair amount of perspiration. That's what happened to me after training. Therefore, I always had a magnesium tablet dissolved in water, and I am still doing this regularly, even if I no longer sweat as much as a few years ago.

The next four weeks, that is week five to eight, you should do your regular cycling six days per week, while increasing the exercise time gradually. I suggest the following increase rhythm:

5th Week: 25 minutes per day of action

6th Week: 30 minutes per day of action

7th Week: 35 minutes per day of action

8th Week: 40 minutes per day of action

Please make sure that you are moving during this training phase always with a heart rate value in the area of fat loss (60 – 70 % MHR).

Your condition will improve considerably, and now it will be possible to achieve a higher average speed with constant resistance. In addition, you will find that your pulse rate will have a sinking tendency.

If you have managed to do these eight weeks consistently, you will find it more and more easy to do your workout. After these eight weeks, the biking will be more and more a matter of course, and your overall well-being will increase.

The ninth and tenth week you will find it no longer troublesome to spend 45 minutes of training on your home trainer or exercise bike.

You will feel fit and at ease.

Your physical condition will have improved significantly in the meantime and you will have reached a level of training that will allow you to extend the endurance training on the rowing machine without any particular effort.

From the eleventh week you should begin, therefore, to include the rowing machine in your workout. Since rowing is however significantly more strenuous than cycling, I recommend the following:

11th Week: 15 minutes of rowing and 30 minutes of cycling

12th Week: 15 minutes of rowing and 30 minutes of cycling

13th Week: 20 minutes of rowing and 25 minutes cycling

14th Week: 25 minutes cycling rowing and 20 minutes

15th Week: 25 minutes cycling rowing and 20 minutes

16th Week: 30 minutes of rowing and 15 minutes cycling

After about four months, your condition will have improved so much that it will be possible for you to pursue rowing for 45 minutes and an additional 15 to 20 minutes of cycling at an average of at least five days per week. I recommend starting the daily training with rowing because it is harder than cycling.

Make sure that during rowing your heart rate continuously moves in the above-defined zone of fat burning.

I consider the rowing training a very effective aerobic exercise, it has a positive effect on the whole body. Then the cycling can be understood as a regeneration phase, since your pulse rate will then be lower than during the rowing. During the last three to five minutes on the bike you should reduce the speed until your pulse rate is significantly reduced, and you can end the endurance training.

Rowing machines with hydraulic resistance will be harder to handle for the first few minutes, because the hydraulic oil needs to warm up before the rowing arms can be moved more easily.

When rowing try to breathe as follows: inhale when moving forward and exhale when you move backward.

For the realization of your endurance training it is very advantageous if you fix a schedule for your daily routine. Our goal should be a 60 minute endurance training in the course of four months. It goes without saying that you work up at least five days a week until you sweat, and that is very healthy! However, to avoid muscle cramps, I recommend a magnesium tablet after your workout.

To keep track of the progress of your personal level of endurance training in the long run, you should note down the respective duration of your sports activities, for example on an agenda. If you can see that you have achieved your weekly target over long period, you will be encouraged to continue in the future!

After six months you will surely feel much fitter fitness and a much improved physical condition and you'll be in a good mood!

If you have "survived" the first half year successfully, then I am sure, you will continue with energy your endurance training for about one hour on the two devices.

Final note about the training

The recommended endurance training has a central importance in the present book for seniors. It is not only the foundation for a significant improvement in fitness, but endurance training is also likely to contribute significantly to improving the overall health.

Medical experts are sure, that there is a specific affinity between blood pressure and physical activity, if the endurance training is exercised for a longer period.

Through systematic endurance training you can thus contribute directly to improving your health, and that's just for the elderly a very important argument to do it.

According to medical assessments on the internet a lot of people suffer from high blood pressure without even noticing. This is especially true with older people. I am therefore convinced that, especially for the age group "60 plus" in the long-term, regular aerobic exercise on stepper, bicycle home trainer or exercise bike and home rowing machine are excellent opportunities to optimize the blood pressure and thus to lay the foundation for getting old in good health.

In the medical field you can also learn that regular exercise has a very positive effect on blood sugar, and the recommended endurance training can surely be seen as a valuable physical activity.

So there is a number of arguments that show that the endurance training can be generally considered as "highly recommended".

These additional health aspects should motivate you to integrate the recommended endurance exercise into your daily routine. You will see that you will find it all the easier to train for an hour on your exercise bike or rowing machine, the longer you practice it!

As your fitness will gradually improve, you will want to increase the resistance on your rowing machine, with a heart rate in the fat burning area. You will spend more and more time on the top of this intensity zone. For a 65 year old senior this amounts to a heart rate from 106 to 108 beats per minute.

When cycling, your heart rate should be more in the lower to middle range of the fat burning area. The pulse rate should therefore not significantly exceed 100 beats. Finish off the last five minutes at low speed accordingly in the health area, for a 65 year old senior that corresponds to about 77 to 92 beats per minute.

In the long run you should row for 45 minutes and cycle for 15 to 30 minutes and this should be done at least five days a week.

If possible, you should swim once a week. Personally because of the different types of exercise that I have been practicing for several years, I have become convinced that varying the different endurance sports for the elderly are highly recommendable because the various body regions are activated.

It also makes sense to spread the various exercises over the week so that almost every day, you do at least one endurance sport, including the walking. And this should be understood as a bottom line: As a senior, you should do an active endurance sport every day for at least 45 minutes.

For me it has become a matter of course to get moving for 45 minutes a day. This daily forty-five minute endurance training requires no special effort. On the contrary, I feel uncomfortable when I cannot do it.

Endurance training is not only very beneficial for the entire heart and circulatory system, for tendons, ligaments and muscles, but it should also have a positive impact on the bones, which is highly beneficial for us elderly!

Basic recommendation SEVEN – how internal balance and mental satisfaction can be achieved

The previous recommendations are mainly aimed at keeping seniors fit and healthy. But it is not enough having a slim, athletic figure!

Only when we find our inner balance and satisfaction, will we cast the basis for a healthy life that makes us happy.

We will learn to be glad about "little things". Then we will have the good fortune of being able to enjoy basic mental satisfaction and happiness and well-being.

Now there is certainly no general formula for reaching basic mental balance and satisfaction.

What is important in this context is, in my view, a fundamentally positive attitude towards life. However, this attitude is missing in many individuals. And where the underlying positive orientation is missing, there is a large risk to plunge into pessimism. In my opinion, a pessimistic orientation provides no access to inner harmony and happiness!

A second way of achieving inner balance lies in the ability to "turn off". In principle, this should actually be easier for us seniors even than for younger ones because we have no more job stress and are less exposed to the daily bustle. Nevertheless, the ability to turn off and relax is not automatic and must be trained.

However, there are several ways to learn to achieve equanimity. Yoga is one for example, as well as other forms of meditation.

An autogenic training as a means of finding inner peace, usually requires the assistance of an experienced teacher.

A sauna can also be very relaxing and thus create true inner peace.

Walking in a park or in a forest can produce genuine inner happiness, created by endorphins! Both my wife and I often have this feeling of happiness when we walk in a natural environment.

Another road to happiness is singing. I am an enthusiastic singer in a choral society and I get a feeling of an internal balance and relaxation singing once a week.

But there are many other social activities that can make you happy and relaxed.

Last, but not least it is our belief in god that makes us find inner peace, harmony and contentment.

A harmonious married life and partnership certainly provide inner peace and contentment. In this regard, in a partnership, each partner is called upon to make his own contribution to conscious harmony balance.

Basic recommendation EIGHT – How to maintain your intellectual fitness

On top of keeping our body in a healthy balance we seniors should take special care that our minds are fit. This intellectual fitness is for me the third important element guaranteeing our staying healthy and fit when we are getting older.

This ultimately means that we seniors need to challenge our minds specifically. There are certainly many different ways of doing that. We must be creative in this regard!

Perhaps various attempts in the field of creativeness must be made to find a viable, long-term concept.

Whatever you opt for, it is essential you find it intellectually demanding. You must make sure that it becomes a personal success. As I am personally interested in physics and astronomy, I sometimes find it hard, for example, to understand Brian Greene, one of the leading physicists in the field of superstring theory, even after a second reading. And yet, it's fascinating challenge! Playing chess sis also a demanding game for me, even if I lose against my chess partner ever so often.

Summary

I recommend the following concept, based on my own experience:

Recommended dietary changes
- Only fruit and a yogurt for supper
- Four times a week no meat
- Neither sausage nor cheese for breakfast
- No sweets
- Restricted alcohol consumption: little beer, little wine

Recommended motion concept

Warming up Exercises
- Two to three times a week, gymnastics for 10 to 15 minutes before starting the endurance training
- Muscle training 2 times per week for about 10 minutes

Endurance Training
- Walking outdoor
        4 times per week for about 40 to 60 minutes
- Rowing (Home rower)

45 minutes a day 5 times per week

- Cycling on exercise bikes or bicycle ergometer

20 - 30 minutes a day 5 times per week

alternating with

- Stepping on stepper

15 - 20 minutes 3 - to 5 times per week

- Swimming

Swimming once a week, 30 minutes

I have been doing these programs for over eight years, and their positive effects can be read at the end of my self-test report.

Suggesting a timetable for the implementation phase

In view of the positive health effects I achieved through these programs I am determined to continue these exercises without expecting to lose more weight, and I am quite happy with my weight loss of about 44 pounds.

I want to continue these programs because I am convinced that they provide for my future life the conditions ensuring lasting health and fitness.

Of course, this does not mean I will be immune to diseases, but nevertheless these activities will contribute to overcome possible diseases more quickly and to prepare for a future in good health. In the long run, we seniors can possibly make sure that we are less burdensome for our family and other people.

I hope that my remarks and recommendations will also induce my fellow seniors to work for leading a healthier life.

As my concept includes several health strategies, I think it is recommendable to proceed gradually, but at the same time, to plan your health programs far ahead.

For this reason I suggest that you start the first steps before reaching the pensionable age. You should focus on the "hard" part of the implementation package namely "moving", your body as much as possible right after your retirement.

One thing is out of the question: Smoking. Stop it as soon as possible! Smoking is more than harmful to your health!

The following chronological approach to a healthier life is recommendable:

Entryphase

You should start your health program about five years before retiring. 60 years of age is a good starting date. Many people at this age are still fully committed to the job, but you should spare some time to do the first steps towards a healthier life.

Begin with the improvement of your immune system through the following activities.

- Walking three times a week for 45 minutes in the fresh air.
- Visit a sauna once a week.

You should begin additionally with the following activities:

- Refrain from eating sausage and cheese for breakfast.
- Eat fruits at least one a day.

This starting phase should cover a period of about two years.

Intensification phase

During this subsequent period starting with your actual retirement I recommend the following activities:

- Reduce the consumption of wine and beer
- Refrain largely from sweets.
- Practice twice a week the proposed gymnastic exercises.
- Practice the recommended strength exercises once or twice a week.

Optimization phase

With the start of retirement, you will have plenty of time available to implement the remaining elements of the action program step by step. In addition, you now have the opportunity to adapt your weekly meal plan to the recommended dietary changes.

Based on my own positive experience I especially appreciate the endurance training as particularly important. However, you have to do that for a long time before enjoying benefits. In this respect, it is therefore necessary to take a long breath.

But your achievements relating to health and fitness will compensate you fully. Your self-esteem will be much greater after two or three years, you will feel good all over, and you will not have any overweight problems!

In addition, you will find that you can sleep well without any tablets and that your bowel movements will function without any medication. Your blood pressure will be lower and your blood sugar will be on good levels. You will be fit and healthy!

But success is 1% inspiration and 99% perspiration. I wish you a lot of success!

OUTLOOK

After I practicing the program recommended by me full nine years, I would like to venture the following prognosis for those who are planning to do it for such a long period:

You will feel completely fit!

You will speak of yourself as being of "robust health" and consulting a doctor will become an exceptional activity!

You have a well-balanced, positive attitude towards life, so that you can look forward to living your future life with confidence!

You will be among those seniors who on to of their own initiative laid the foundation for an excellent future. And here we will find a most rewarding challenge! Due to the growing longevity of seniors our lives after retirement can still last remarkably long. The longer we live, the more important it is, to stay healthy and fit as long as possible. And in this regard we have to become active!

A healthy diet and regular physical exercise are exciting prospects, to help prevent long-time illnesses, especially of the heart and circulatory troubles. So there is a lot we can do to stay fit and healthy. Let's do it now!

VITA

The author was born in 1941 in Heilbronn / Germany. When his father was killed in war in Russia, the mother moved with him as an infant to the grandparents in the Black Forest. After finishing High School, he studied economics and earned his degree at the University of Munich. In the following years he held several management positions in industry and worked as an independent business consultant for small and medium-sized enterprises. With 64 years he ended his career and retired.

Shortly thereafter, he visited the doctor to perform a health check and it turned out that his blood pressure was clearly too high. His doctor said that either he has to take pills for the rest of his life or his excessive weight has to be reduced by at least 33 pounds. The author chose the weight loss. By following the diet and training plan developed by him he managed to reduce his weight by about 44 pounds.

Since friends insisted several times to learn about the secrets of his success, he decided about 4 years ago to write his first book in German. Two years later, an extended revision of the German book was released. Now, in the age of 73, he releases his first English-language book titled;

"You can do what I did: lose weight, improve your health, stay fit!